Paleo Slow Cooker Cookbook

Easy Everyday Recipes for Busy Moms

Just to say "Thank you" for purchasing this book.

I want to give you a Free Gift!

GO TO PALEOLUV.COM TO GRAB YOUR FREE GIFT.

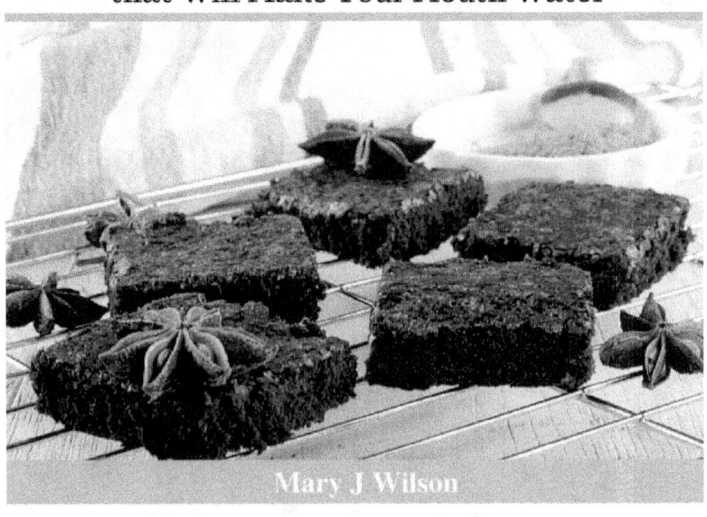

Delectable
PALEO
Desserts
A Dozen Quick and Easy Paleo Desserts
that Will Make Your Mouth Water

Mary J Wilson

Contents

Disclaimer

The recipes provided in this report are for informational purposes only and are not intended to provide dietary advice. A medical practitioner should be consulted before making any changes in diet. Additionally, recipe cooking times may require adjustment depending on age and quality of appliances. Readers are strongly urged to take all precautions to ensure ingredients are fully cooked in order to avoid the dangers of foodborne viruses. The recipes and suggestions provided in this book are solely the opinion of the author. The author and publisher do not take any responsibility for any consequences that may result due to following the instructions provided in this book.

INTRODUCTION

Clean, delicious food, slow-cooked to perfection and healthy to boot is what we all want to be cooking in our kitchens. But as a busy mom, it can sometimes seem like a nearly impossible task to delve into some home cooking, let alone make that cooking something nutritious and delicious too.

Luckily, there is a solution to this challenge. It's called *Paleo Slow Cooker Cookbook: Everyday Easy Recipes for Busy Moms.* There is a way you can eat healthy and create those fresh meals in your very own kitchen without spending ridiculous amounts of time doubled over a stove.

We've combined a diet and a cooking method that's going to make your life a whole lot easier and your waistline a whole lot slimmer with *Paleo Slow Cooker Cookbook: Everyday Easy Recipes for Busy Moms.*

The Paleo Diet is all about returning to eating the way our ancestors did thousands of years ago. Far before mass production and the industrial revolution, there was a little thing called nature that gave us everything we needed for optimum health.

Nature's table included an array of fruits, vegetables, nuts, and animal proteins. Foods were meant to be simple, eaten raw or cooked over a quick fire. These are the types of foods our bodies were designed to break down naturally, and that's why these are the same types of foods that leave us feeling revitalized, energetic, and healthy.

These types of foods that nature provides don't just leave you feeling great, but they leave you looking great too. The nutrients and antioxidants found in Paleo foods put a shine in your hair, a glow in your face, and give an overall radiance to your being.

Essentially, you need to stay away from foods that require a ton of processing to be edible. If you were meant to eat those things, your body should be able to break it down without the assistance of machines. This is why the Paleo diet eliminates breads and cereals, sugary treats, and processed snack foods. Additionally, dairy is also eliminated on Paleo.

People new to the Paleo lifestyle often feel intimidated because they assume the diet has to be hard, and in turn they're likely to have to spend all sorts of time concocting strange recipes. And although you can concoct whatever recipes you wish, it doesn't have to be hard.

Drumroll….

Enter the slow cooker.

Delicious food, easy-to-prepare, and loaded with everything you need to be healthy and super slim IS possible, AND it's not going to cost you crazy dinero to achieve the fantasy.

The slow cooker has been around for decades, but it still feels like a modern miracle in any kitchen. All you need to do is pop your ingredients into the magic pot, set it, and forget about it until the timer goes off. We've created breakfast, lunch, dinner, and even snacks that you can make right in your slow cooker for all kinds of one-pot happiness.

For breakfast, you're going to want to check out the absolutely delicious Avocado and Zucchini Fritsters and the Open Face

Breakfast Sandwich. If you've got a hankering for something on the sweet tip, check out the Coconut Porridge.

For Lunch, try the divine Cuban sandwich or maybe the wickedly easy Overnight Chili. For dinner you can let yourself indulge in the tastes of the East with a little Chicken Curry dish or for something with a little zing, check out the Coconut Beef with Lime.

The Snacks section will help you get through those times when you've got a hankering for something in between meals, but all you can find are donuts and cupcakes. The Snacks section includes Jalapeno Pops and a gorgeous Carne Asada dip you're surely get addicted to.

All of the recipes provided in the *Paleo Slow Cooker Cookbook: Everyday Easy Recipes for Busy Moms* are meant to make your life a lot simpler because being a mom is a full time job. The dishes are supremely easy to make with ingredients that should be easy for you to source locally.

Additionally, the kids are going to love some of the flavors we've put together. They're so good, they don't even taste healthy!

Enjoy sharing the *Paleo Slow Cooker Cookbook: Everyday Easy Recipes for Busy Moms* with your family. We hope it helps you have one less thing you've got to concern yourself with between the hundreds of other things you're doing all day long.

Happy Sloooow—cooking!

BREAKFAST

The Open-Faced Sausage Sandwich

Serves: 4
Total Time: 7 hours

Ingredients

1 lb sausage meat

4 pastured eggs

2 green bell peppers, seeded, chopped

1 medium white onion, chopped

½ tsp salt

½ tsp black pepper

Directions

- Place sausage meat in bottom of slow cooker.
- Combine eggs with bell pepper, onion, salt, black pepper, mix.
- Pour eggs on top of sausage.

- o Turn slow cooker to low and cook overnight for 7 hours.

- o Slice into quarters and serve.

- o If you need to take it to go, slice into eighths so you can make a sandwich with two of the slices.

Nutrition (g)

Calories 475

Fat 36

Carbs 7

Sugars 4

Protein 29

Coconut Porridge

Serves: 4
Total Time: 7 hours

Ingredients

1 cup coconut flakes

¼ cup flaxseed

½ cup walnuts, chopped

1 cup coconut milk

½ cup water

4 Medjool Dates

½ tsp cinnamon

Directions

- Combine ingredients in a 4-quart slow cooker.
- Cook on low overnight for 7 hours.

Nutrition (g)

Calories 403

Fat 32

Carbs 26

Sugars 17

Protein 8

Spinach Quiche

Serves: 4
Total Time: 7 hours

Ingredients

1 lb spinach, washed and chopped

1 medium onion, chopped

1 cup almonds, chopped

4 pastured eggs

½ tsp salt

½ tsp black pepper

Coconut oil

Directions

- Combine almonds with 2 tablespoons of coconut oil.

- Place almond mixture in the bottom of a medium slow cooker.

- Crack eggs into a bowl, whisk, and add salt and black pepper, mix.

- Place spinach and onion on top of almonds in slow cooker.

o   Pour your eggs over the top and cook on low for 7 hours.

Nutrition (g)

Calories 264

Fat 20

Carbs 13

Sugars 3

Protein 15

Cauliflower Hash

Serves: 4
Total Time: 4 hours

Ingredients

1 medium cauliflower

1 lb low sodium ham

½ tsp black pepper

½ tsp salt

Coconut oil

Directions

- o Grate cauliflower and mix with salt and black pepper.
- o Coat a medium slow cooker with coconut oil.
- o Place your cauliflower in slow-cooker, add ham on top.
- o Cook on high for 4 hours.

Nutrition (g)

Calories 137

Fat 2

Carbs 10

Sugars 4

Protein 21

Avocado and Zucchini Fritters

Serves: 4
Total Time: 7 hours

Ingredients

1 avocado, pitted, skin-removed

5 zucchinis, peeled, grated

2 eggs

2 tbsp coconut flour

1 tbsp fresh dill

½ tsp salt

½ tsp black pepper

Directions

- Whisk eggs in a bowl.

- Squeeze excess liquid from zucchini.

- Combine zucchini with eggs, coconut flour, dill, salt and black pepper, let the mixture sit for 5 minutes.

- Place zucchini into slow cooker, place avocado slices on top.

- Cook on low for 7 hours.

Nutrition (g)

Calories 193

Fat 13

Carbs 16

Sugars 5

Protein 8

LUNCH

Pork and Apple Stew

Serves: 6
Total Time: 7 hours

Ingredients

2 lb pork tenderloin

1 sweet potato, peeled

1 apple, peeled, cored

1 onion, diced

4 cloves garlic, minced

¼ tsp rosemary

½ tsp salt

½ tsp black pepper

Extra virgin olive oil

Directions

- o   Slice pork tenderloin into 1" cubes.
- o   Slice sweet potato and apple into 1" cubes.

- o   Coat slow cooker with a little olive oil.

- o   Heat 2 tablespoons extra virgin olive oil in skillet.

- o   Add pork and brown.

- o   Place pork in slow cooker, add remaining ingredients.

- o   Cook on low for 7 hours.

Nutrition (g)

Calories 300

Fat 10

Carbs 11

Sugars 5

Protein 40

The Cuban Sandwich

Serves: 1
Total Time: 10 minutes

Ingredients

3 slices high-quality cured ham

2 slices slow-roasted pork (recipe in dinner the section of this book)

3 slices pickles

¼ avocado, pitted, skin-removed, sliced

½ tsp organic mustard

2 lettuce leaves

Directions

- o Turn on a sandwich grill.
- o Lay your lettuce leaves on a flat surface.
- o Spread mustard on your lettuce leaf.
- o Layer ham, pickles, pork and avocado.
- o Roll up lettuce wrap, place wrap in the grill.
- o And grill for a few minutes.

Nutrition (g)

Calories 411

Fat 28

Carbs 9

Sugar 1

Protein 32

Tilapia in Coconut Sauce

Serves: 4
Total Time: 7 hours

Ingredients

4 x 4oz tilapia filets

1 green onion, chopped

1 tbsp ginger, grated

1 cup coconut milk

½ tsp paprika

½ tsp cumin

½ tsp salt

½ tsp black pepper

Coconut oil

Directions

- Lightly coat a medium slow cooker with coconut oil.

- Place tilapia filets in slow cooker.

- Combine coconut milk with green onion, ginger, salt, black pepper, paprika, cumin and pour over filets.

- o Cook on low overnight for 7 hours.

- o Enjoy with a green salad.

Nutrition (g)

Calories 293

Fat 18

Carbs 5

Sugars 2

Protein 31

Overnight Chili

Serves: 4
Total Time: 7 hours

Ingredients

1-1/2 lb grass-fed ground beef

1 onion, chopped

4 cloves garlic, minced

1 carrot, chopped

1 celery stalk, chopped

1 cup tomato puree

1 cup organic chicken stock

¾ tsp cumin

¾ tsp oregano

1 tsp salt

1 tsp black pepper

Coconut Oil

Directions

- Heat 2 tbsp coconut oil in a skillet over medium heat.

- o Add onion and sauté until translucent, add garlic and sauté for 30 seconds.

- o Add ground beef, sauté of 5 minutes.

- o Place all ingredients in a medium slow cooker and turn to low.

- o Cook overnight for 7 hours and lunch will be ready in the morning.

Nutrition (g)

Calories 303

Fat 19

Carbs 12

Sugars 5

Protein 23

Chicken with Tomato Basil Spaghetti

Serves: 1
Total Time: 4 hours

Ingredients

16 oz chicken breasts

1 medium spaghetti squash

1 cup tomato sauce

6 basil leaves, chopped

4 cloves garlic, minced

1 medium onion, minced

salt

black pepper

Coconut oil

Directions

- Brush medium slow cooker with coconut oil.

- Chop squash into quarters, remove rind, brush with coconut oil, sprinkle with ½ tsp salt and ½ tsp black pepper, and place in slow cooker.

- Top squash with garlic cloves, onion, basil leaves, tomato sauce.

- o Brush chicken breasts with coconut oil and sprinkle with a little salt.

- o Place chicken strips on top of everything.

- o Cook on high for four hours.

Nutrition (g)

Calories 295

Fat 10

Carbs 15

Sugars 4

Protein 35

DINNER

Beefy Red Bell Lasagna

Serves: 6
Total Time: 7 hours

Ingredients

1 lb pastured ground beef

2 red bell peppers, seeded, sliced

1 medium head cauliflower

4 cups tomato puree

1 cup organic chicken stock

1 bay leaf

½ tsp oregano

½ tsp black pepper

1 tsp salt

Coconut oil

Directions

- Chop cauliflower into florets.

- Place florets into food processor and pulse until you've got rice like granules.

- Heat 2 tbsp coconut oil in skillet over medium heat.

- Brown beef, set aside.

- Brush a medium slow cooker with coconut oil.

- Combine tomato puree, chicken stock with oregano, black pepper, salt, and bay leaf.

- Place a third of your cauliflower in the bottom of the slow cooker, next layer 1/2 your beef mixture, 1/2 red bell pepper, 1/3 of your tomato sauce.

- Repeat and top with remaining cauliflower and tomato sauce.

- Cover slow cooker, turn to low, and cook for 7 hours.

Nutrition (g)

Calories 404

Fat 19

Carbs 34

Sugars 18

Protein 29

Curry Chicken Breast

Serves: 4
Total Time: 7 hours

Ingredients

1 lb chicken breast, cubed

1 onion, diced

6 cloves garlic, minced

1 green bell pepper, seeded, diced

2 tbsp tomato paste

1 tsp curry powder

½ tsp cumin powder

½ tsp paprika

½ tsp salt

½ tsp black pepper

Coconut oil

Directions

- Slice chicken breasts into 1" cubes.
- Coat a medium slow cooker with coconut oil.
- Place all of your ingredients into a slow cooker and cook on low for 7 hours overnight.

Nutrition (g)

Calories 234

Fat 5

Carbs 8

Sugars 4

Protein 38

Garlicky Lamb Meatballs

Serves: 4
Total Time: 7 hours

Ingredients

1 ½ lb grass-fed lamb

1 egg

1 tbsp coconut flour

1 tbsp cumin

1 tbsp garlic powder

1 tbsp onion powder

1 tbsp oregano

2 tbsp salt

1 tbsp black pepper

Extra virgin olive oil

Directions

- Whisk eggs.
- Combine all ingredients in a bowl.
- Preheat oven to 350 degrees Farenheit.
- Shape mixture into 1 ½ " meatballs.

o Place meatballs in slow cooker and cook on low for 7 hours.

Nutrition (g)

Calories 402

Fat 23

Carbs 7

Sugars 1

Protein 22

Coconut Beef with Lime

Serves: 4
Total Time: 4 hours

Ingredients

1 ½ lb flank steak

2 green onions, chopped

1 tbsp grated ginger

1 red bell pepper, seeded, sliced

1 cup coconut milk

1 tbsp lemongrass, chopped

1 bay leaf, ground

1 cup water

Coconut oil

Directions

- o   Slice flank steak into ½" strips.
- o   Combine all ingredients in medium slow cooker.
- o   Cook on high for 4 hours.

Nutrition (g)

Calories 405

Fat 27

Carbs 7

Sugars 4

Protein 34

Chicken and Sweet Potato Casserole

Serves: 6
Total Time: 7 hours

Ingredients

12 skinless, boneless chicken thighs.

3 sweet potatoes, peeled

1 cup organic chicken stock

1 tsp rosemary

1 tsp black pepper

1 tsp salt

Extra Virgin Olive Oil

Directions

- Slice sweet potatoes into ¼" slices.
- Coat medium slow cooker with coconut oil.
- Combine salt, black pepper, rosemary, and 2 tablespoons of extra virgin olive oil.
- Rub chicken thighs with rosemary rub.
- Place 1/3 of sweet potatoes on bottom of slow cooker.
- Place four chicken thighs on top, layer sweet potato, chicken thighs, repeat.
- Pour chicken stock over top.
- Cover and cook on low for 7 hours.

Nutrition (g)

Calories 492

Fat 11

Carbs 56

Sugars 1

Protein 41

SNACKS

Creamy Eggplant Dip

Serves: 4
Total Time: 4 hours

Ingredients

4 Chinese eggplants

1 cup coconut milk

½ tsp cumin

½ tsp oregano

1 red onion, minced

4 cloves garlic, minced

Coconut oil

Extra virgin olive oil

Directions

- Coat a medium slow cooker with extra virgin oil.

- Pierce eggplants in several spots and place into slow cooker.

- o Add onions, garlic, and spices into slow cooker, and drizzle with 4 tablespoons olive oil.

- o Cook on high for 4 hours, remove eggplant, peel, and crush.

- o Return eggplant to slow cooker along with coconut milk and cook for another hour on high.

- o Mix well and serve.

Nutrition (g)

Calories 254

Fat 17

Carbs 26

Sugars 13

Protein 5

Jalapeno Pops

Serves: 4
Total Time: 4 hours

Ingredients

12 jalapenos

½ cup walnuts, crushed

¼ cup coconut milk

½ tsp paprika

½ tsp salt

½ tsp black pepper

Coconut oil

1 cup water

Directions

- o Place walnuts in food processor along with 3 tablespoons coconut milk, salt, black pepper, paprika and mix until fairly smooth.

- o Slice jalapenos in half, remove seeds.

- o Scoop a little bit of the walnut mixture into each jalapeno half.

- o Place jalapenos in your slow cooker and cook on high for four hours.

Nutrition (g)

Calories 155

Fat 14

Carbs 5

Sugars 2

Protein 5

Mushroom Bites

Serves: 4
Total Time: 4 hours

Ingredients

20 button mushrooms

4 cloves garlic

½ cup parsley, stemmed, chopped

¼ cup organic chicken stock

¼ cup ghee

1 tsp salt

1 tsp black pepper

Directions

- o   Melt ghee in saucepan over medium heat, add garlic and sauté for 20 seconds.
- o   Place mushrooms and parsley in slow cooker, add garlic ghee and mix.
- o   Cook on high for 4 hours.

Nutrition (g)

Calories 138

Fat 13

Carbs 4

Sugars 2

Protein 3

Peppered Carrot

Serves: 4
Total Time: 3 hours

Ingredients

16 carrots, peeled

½ tsp black pepper

1 tsp hot chili pepper

1 tsp salt

Directions

- o Slice carrot into ½" thick matchsticks.
- o Combine carrot with spices.
- o Place carrot in slow cooker and cook on high for 3 hours.

Nutrition (g)

Calories

Fat

Carbs

Sugars

Protein

Carne Asada Dip

Serves: 6
Total Time: 7 hours

Ingredients

2 lb flank steak

½ avocado, pitted, peeled, sliced

1 medium onion, diced

1 red bell pepper, diced

2 ancho chilies stemmed and seeded.

5 cloves garlic, minced

1 tsp cumin

1 tsp oregano

1 tsp paprika

1 orange, juiced

3 limes, juiced

Coconut oil

Directions

- Place all ingredients, save avocado, in slow cooker and cook on low for 7 hours.

- o Top with avocado and serve with veggies or dehydrated vegetable chips.

Nutrition (g)

Calories 390

Fat 18

Carbs 8

Sugars 5

Protein 43

CONCLUSION

Of course you want to ensure your family is eating well, which in turn means they are getting all the nutrition they need to excel in life. But sometimes switching your family over to a healthier way of eating is easier said than done. Old, familiar tastes die hard and letting go of comfort food can be anything but comfortable.

The great thing about the Paleo lifestyle is that it makes switching to healthy living very easy. With Paleo, you're still eating a lot of the foods you enjoy. In fact, some of those foods that you thought were bad for you are actually good, so you can eat without guilt! Namely, eating certain types of fat is not going to make you fat. Your body needs fat for numerous functions, and it is fat that's going to keep your skin supple and young.

The most difficult part for most people when switching to Paleo is letting go of those pesky carbohydrates. In the Paleo Slow Cooker Recipes for Busy Moms, we've made it easy to replace the carbs with equally satisfying low-carb substitutes that pack all of the flavor and texture you want without the sugars that can poison your body.

Cooking nutritious and delicious meals for your family doesn't have to be difficult. In fact, as we've learned with Paleo Slow Cooker Recipes for Busy Moms, it can be as easy as one, two, done. The most difficult part of home cooking for most busy moms is the time that it takes to plan and prep meals, and that's where the slow cooker comes in.

The slow cooker method is very forgiving, and moreover, it also produces tasty, comforting meals. All you need to do is get your ingredients ready, toss them in a single pot – the slow cooker – and you're done. You spend mere minutes in the prep work, and the slow cooker does all the rest, and you don't have a ton of pots and pans to clean up after!

The Paleo Slow Cooker Recipes for Busy Moms is designed to help you live a simple, clean, home-cooked kind of life without any of the fuss. Enjoy the recipes and take advantage of all that time you're saving by spending it on the people and things most important in your life.

Happy Slow Cooking!

I Need Your Help!

Please take a minute out of your busy schedule to leave a review. Your review will let readers know what to expect and what you liked about this book. I am looking forward to reading your review!
Thank you so much for your feedback!

Go the following URL to leave a review

https://www.amazon.com/review/create-review#